Grigori Grabovoi

Educational System of Grigori Grabovoi

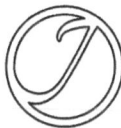

Jeletzky publishing, Hamburg 2011

Jelezky publishing, Hamburg

www.jelezky-media.com

1st Edition

First English Edition, September 2011

© 2011 English Language Edition

Dimitri Eletski, Hamburg (Publisher)

English Translation: Lingua Communications Translation Services, USA

This translation has been done from the Russian text transcribed from the recording of the author´s live seminar, conducted in Moscow on February 7, 2000

For further information on the contents of this book contact:

SVET centre, Hamburg, Germany,

www.svet-centre.eu

ISBN: 978-3-943110-15-9

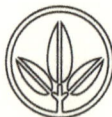

According to the responses we have received, the contents of this book have helped many people. We are confident that this will continue to be the case.

Nonetheless, we would like to point out that the techniques of Grigori Grabovoi are mental methods for the guidance of events in one's life. These methods are dependent upon one's personal spiritual development. Because we are dealing with topics relating to one's health, we give this express notice that such influence is not a "therapy" in the conventional sense of the word and is therefore not intended to limit or replace professional medical care.

When in doubt, follow the directions of your doctor or a therapist or pharmacist whom you trust! (When following conventional methods, you must expect to get conventional results.)

Jelelezky Publishing/SVET center, Hamburg

Educational System of Grigori Grabovoi

Edition: 2011-1, 04.09.2011

Educational System of Grigori Grabovoi

My system of education is based on the fact that I provide knowledge even before a person is born. Therefore my system of education is based on concentration and on the transfer of knowledge even before the person is born. This can be done by the parents of the baby to be born, and therefore grandparents and, in principle, any people who are in a position to consider that someone is about to have a baby, a new person.

This system of education includes several stages.

The first stage is through concentration on infinity, that is, on infinite time and space before the birth of the person – to concentrate on the first thought: *let him be born, creatively develop and give eternity to the world.*

Having concentrating the thought three years prior to birth, to effect the following mental formula: *the person who is born must live joyously, happily and surrounded by love.*

After concentrating the thought one year prior to the birth of the person, it is necessary to mentally state: *this person will always be happy and he will bring happiness and love to others and himself. He will always be well provided for and he will not be lacking in anything.* This thought needs to be mentally led through the point which is the three-year point, that is, the one I have mentioned as occurring three years prior to birth; then mentally take it through infinity, by mental action sort of bring this event through, and in fact bring through in reality all the infinite information prior to birth and then transfer it to the infinite information after birth and bring it directly to the point of birth of the person; at first – to the point of his conception. This way that action on concentration performed one year prior to birth,

5

that is, it is expressed as movement of thought along a number of points. Therefore, by a succession of simple actions it is possible to space these points out along a straight line; I will show that as Figure 1.

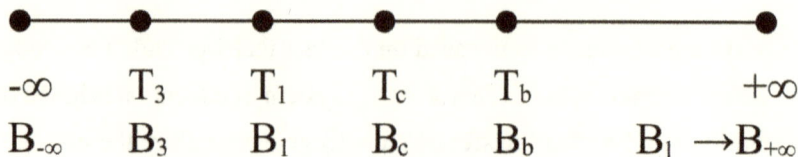

$$\bullet \quad\quad \bullet \quad\quad \bullet \quad\quad \bullet \quad\quad \bullet \quad\quad\quad\quad\quad \bullet$$

$-\infty$	T_3	T_1	T_c	T_b	$+\infty$
$B_{-\infty}$	B_3	B_1	B_c	B_b	$B_1 \rightarrow B_{+\infty}$

Fig. 1. Before and after birth

Along the straight line, that is, the point of infinity, negative infinity $(-\infty)$ is located on the left, then it is followed, that is, by the point of conception, I write it as T_c – indicating the point of conception, then the point at one year prior to birth – T_1, and point T_3 – three years prior to birth. And, that is, on the right side there will be the point of positive infinity $(+\infty)$.

This way, when I am saying that it is necessary to mentally work with the point of conception – for example, take it – when I said that it is necessary to lead the thought from point one to point three through negative infinity, positive infinity and then to the point of conception – it is possible to do that even along the same straight line. That is: to concentrate on point T_c, the point of conception and already from there to transition to point one, having formulated the thought, which I stated; to lead it mentally, that is sort of along the straight line to point T_c, then to point negative infinity and then to the point positive infinity and then again to point T_c.

Here there is one more point, which is called the point of birth, that is, and therefore the way it works that if you keep working then the transfer is effected as the transfer of the concept of points into the concept of time. That is – and I already transfer them into concept B_b – time of birth; B_c –

time of conception; B_1, B_2, – time one, time two, and it comes to $B_{-\infty}$ – time of negative infinity and $B_{+\infty}$ – time of positive infinity. This way we have, that is, altogether four points, the meaningful ones, that is, an actual four points that indicate the following:

- three years prior to birth, that is point B_3, three years prior to birth;
- B_1 – one year prior to birth;
- B_c – this is the point of conception;
- B_b – point of birth; and
- $+\infty$ – positive infinity, point $-\infty$ – negative infinity.

There is also the concept of point, the concept of special time, – I will introduce the time of life. So, the time of life must aim for the time of infinity; that means, that the meaning of these actions should be expressed in the fact that life has become infinite, that is – it must aim for positive infinity ($+\infty$). Therefore, this is not signified as a point anymore, but is an infinite element.

Each action – the one, that is, which exists here in this system, my system of education – is aimed at providing concepts of infinite life, infinite creation; and therefore initially it is important to proceed from what this technology promotes specifically in this direction. In doing so all these actions can be implemented with respect to any person regardless of how old that person is at this time. That is, this is to be used not only for future newborns, but can also be applied to all people already living; but in that case it means simply that these concentrations need to be directed to the living person in question, in order to ensure his development towards infinite life and good health, happiness and love.

That is, now I am about to proceed to speak about, that is, actions, concentrations, which need to be present at the point of conception.

That is, in the beginning I will point out the monthly rhythm. That is, in the first month – that is, after the time of conception already – it is necessary to concentrate on trees, animals and people; and to mentally remember one law and transmit that law to the person who is now in the process of development. The law is as follows: *that all the elements of the world, all particles – they connect to each other, and as they connect, they grow.* That is the formula that needs to be mentally sent to the newborn. That is done during the first month.

That is, then there is the second month of development after the point of conception, that is after the actual conception time. There will be a schematic shown in Figure 2, and it is also along a straight line.

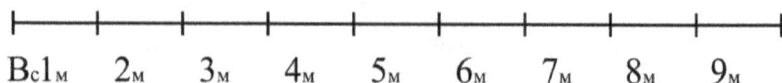

$$\vdash\!\!-\!\!+\!\!-\!\!+\!\!-\!\!+\!\!-\!\!+\!\!-\!\!+\!\!-\!\!+\!\!-\!\!+\!\!-\!\!+\!\!-\!\dashv$$

$B_c1_M \quad 2_M \quad 3_M \quad 4_M \quad 5_M \quad 6_M \quad 7_M \quad 8_M \quad 9_M$

Fig. 2. Nine months of antenatal development

That is, there is the interval of the first month; and then it is followed by the second month already. During the second month it is necessary to mentally broadcast to the developing fetus, the developing person, that *the world is set up in such a way that when you are thinking, then matter becomes organized; and when he starts thinking, matter will become organized as well.*

During the third month after the time of conception it is necessary to broadcast to the future newborn, that is, that *you are part of the world and he is a part of the world, but that he is also an independent part of the world at the same time and because of that he has to think about himself as an independent, separate part of the world.*

The fourth month after, that is, the time of conception it is already necessary to periodically send the thought to the newborn – the future new-born, that is – the developing person, that *he is an individual personality that has started developing already prior to the time of conception, that he has appeared not out of infinity, but has formed himself on his own, and therefore his soul and body are eternal.*

During the fifth month after the time of conception it is necessary to periodically mentally send the following formula: that *the future newborn must already now have a clear understanding as to how he will creatively develop the world and himself in a constructive way.*

During the sixth month after the time, during the sixth month after the time of conception it is necessary to periodically send the following formula. I would like to point out to you here that the concept of "periodically send" means simply to state mentally to the future child as frequently as possible and therefore the more frequently you do it, the better. That is, during the sixth month it is necessary to convey mentally to the future new-born, that *he is responsible for the parents, for phenomena in the surrounding world, that he himself builds up all events and that he must understand that studying all sciences must take place taking into consideration the knowledge, which he receives now; that all sciences will be transformed in his own mind and acquire the meaning which he has placed there from the very beginning in his development; he must understand, that infinity, which existed before him and which exists after, can be combined,* that is what you just transmit as a mental impulse, say in the way you see in Figure 1 – connect the point of negative infinity, the time of negative infinity, positive time, or simply superimpose the symbol B minus over B plus during that sixths month and so it will be that he is already creating life in a harmonized way.

That is, during the seventh month – in the seventh month it is already

9

necessary to convey the mental formula that *the person is responsible for all his actions and he is a mature personality.* It is necessary and mandatory to transmit that he is a mature personality in the same way also at the time of conception. He must openly and clearly recognize, that on the basis of the eternal existing soul he could perceive himself also as a developed personality at the initial moment in the same way as at seven months.

Then at eight months it is necessary to mentally inform him that a *person is born for the purpose of giving birth to others, creating together with others, resurrecting others if they passed away earlier and not allowing others to die; and also not to die.* This is achieved by the fact that point B positive infinity is mentally conveyed to him as the point for which he must strive.

During the ninth month, – during the ninth month it is necessary to mentally broadcast, that *he is an adult person, that he is already capable of breathing, that he can move freely and be equal to others. That is he must get used to the point of birth.*

Then there is the next stage, shown in Figure 3 – this is the moment of birth.

Therefore, Figure 1 indicates a scheme – this is prior to birth, before birth and after; Figure 2, that is, nine months of development – antenatal development, nine months of antenatal development. And if the child already developed earlier, and it was born at earlier than nine months, still it is necessary to speak as if he had developed at the specified antenatal level, that is, there is no difference here. And the only thing is that if he had been born earlier, it would have been possible to superimpose the subsequent period of time over the current one. That is, let's suppose that he was to be born at seven months, then the subsequent formulas, which cover months eight and nine, need to be spoken at the same time.

Figure 3 is called the „Moment or period of birth".

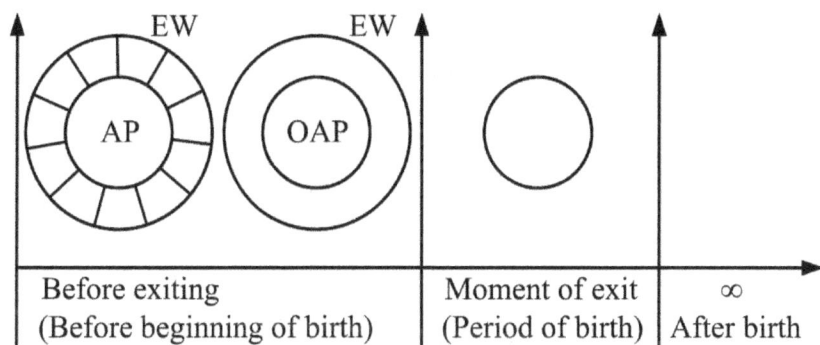

Before exiting (Before beginning of birth)	Moment of exit (Period of birth)	∞ After birth

Fig. 3. Moment of birth (period of birth)

In order to control this period, this moment, from the standpoint of infinite life, the following actions are necessary: to visualize mentally, that the child is connected by infinite connections while he is in the antenatal period. I will show it on the figure as this symbol **AP** – antenatal period, that is, as a sphere; and this sphere has infinite connections, they are like small lines, that is, which transition to another sphere and this signifies the entire world. That is now it is necessary to imagine that there are two spheres. The first sphere is antenatal development, and the second is the whole world, and there is the connection between them. So it is necessary to convey absolutely clearly to the person who is being born that *antenatal development transitions to the next sphere, which is not different from the sphere that he already had, but it is different only in terms of connections to the outside sphere.* That is, it is necessary to have him understand very clearly that those connections here, which in the form of lines were going from the

11

sphere **"AP"** to the sphere that is already here, I will write **"OAP"** –
that is the period outside the antenatal period, that is when the person
is already born and, that is, the external spheres are preserved in the
same way, that is what I am going to indicate as **"EW"** – the external
world; **"EW"** is the external world – this is the external sphere, and
just clearly imagine that now, if before there were certain lines that
connected **AP**, then now this sphere is located within the sphere **EW**,
which is the period outside of antenatal development, when the person
is already born. This needs to be conveyed to him clearly before the
person leaves the body of the mother, that is – before the moment of
exit. It needs to be planted in his attention before the moment of exit.

And then there will be subsequent knowledge, here before the moment
of exit they are sort of divided, for example, by points, and then, that is, at
the moment of exit. The moment of exit needs to be visualized clearly, that
the whole world can be imagined as a sphere and mentally this world can
be passed into his hands. Mentally give it to him right at the very moment
of exit or period of exit, and then the next stage will occur later, that is, in
positive infinity. Here one needs to imagine an open infinite space, that is
the infinite plane, infinite space, and feel that the child is located there, that
the child is located in that infinite space. In fact it looks as though you see
the child in an infinite area. So those actions which, that is, occurred, these
actions indicate that the child is aware of the world before the event occurs
and therefore, when you combine with that awareness you thus are helping
the childbirth, and when you transfer the child into infinity then he feels
comfortable and normal there. So in that entire technology it is important
to work mentally as frequently as possible, and it is possible to work up
to the moment of birth in advance there – as much time as you want in
advance. It is possible to work till the moment of birth over the area that I

have placed in Figure 3.

Now, that is, further on in Figure 4, I am showing the transfer of information by the days after birth.

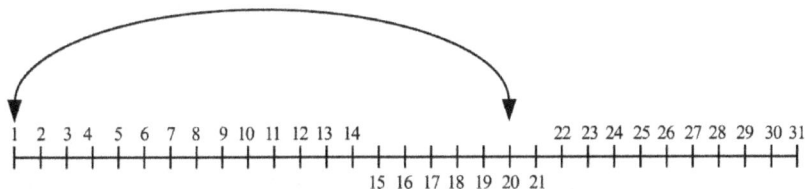

Fig. 4. Information by days after birth

That is, on the first day of birth it is necessary to convey the thought that the *world is eternal.*

Secondly, on the second day after birth, it is necessary to convey the thought that the *world is eternal, but at the same time it changes, it moves and everything in the world develops.*

On the third day after birth, it is necessary to convey that this is why it is eternal – because it moves and develops.

On the fourth day after birth, it is necessary to concentrate on the child and tell him several times in a row that *he has to repeat everything that you told him on the first three days after birth.*

On the fifth day after birth, it is necessary to tell the child mentally that he has to *convey to you mentally what he sees as the world, how he understands the world, and convey to him your love, affection, and happiness that you have in your eyes and soul and give him an opportunity to feast on all the realities that arise from the juxtaposition of the five planes of the world.*

On the sixth day after birth, you need to let the child think independently about how he must convey to you knowledge, information and talk

13

about situations.

On the seventh day after birth, you need to tell the child that *this is the number seven of the day after his birth and this number is sent from above and that there is a Creator who created everything; that father and mother were created by the Creator and that the child himself can also be a Creator, if he understands now how the Creator created this number seven, how he created the world.*

On the eighth day after birth, you must mentally convey that *your child is an element of eternity, that he is infinite, and that if you put a figure eight down on its side you will have infinity, and if you transform the eight into zero, you can transform the entire numerical axis.* That is, you must have him learn to count, let's say, based on the transformation of symbols through a mental transfer of information, and in this way he must understand how one builds his body through a combination of elements. That is, as soon as he feels the way you can, for example, separate an eight and receive a zero, if you look at it sort of from the other side, from the side of the numerical axis, then it may be that it is a zero that is just bent that way. That is, so it goes that he has transformed all elements to zero, and will have approximately that picture, that he can see the transformation of numbers, that is he can transform any matter into anything else, that is, to re-create himself.

On the ninth day, you must say that *he is an individual personality, who unites all the elements of the world, and that he himself creates the world and therefore he is unique, and very wonderful, very happy, and praise him in every way.*

On the tenth day after birth, you need to say that *the number eight which he has converted into zero, that is, it has been converted into one. That is – after the transformation of eight into zero, we received one.* Using this example you need to explain how the world is born, how all the connections in the world occur and how he must be aware of that, among other things.

On the eleventh day after birth, you need to say that *the child should look around using his mental gaze and become aware of himself as a creative personality who is helping mom and dad.*

On the twelfth day after birth, it is necessary to say to the child first in words, and then mentally, that he is the best. That is, first you need to say to the child: *" You are the best one ", and then say the same thing mentally, and do this several times.*

On the thirteenth day after birth, it is necessary to allow the child to play as much as possible with some objects. Give him a pacifier to hold in his hand, etc.

On the fourteenth day after birth, it is necessary to rub the child's feet or, for example, rub them mentally. Also, it is possible on the thirteenth day after birth to mentally place more material objects in the child's hands and, that is, to say two words: "Yes, no, yes, no". This way by repeating it, but not more than 10 times – no more than ten times, and look how he reacts to your next phrase. If you say right away: "Light is the world", the child may react, for example, in some way, but if you say the phrase: "The world is light", he may react differently. This can be all said mentally. And depending on how he reacts, if he reacts openly, that is, emotionally to "Light is the world", – and the reaction may appear in the course of the day, not immediately – then you must – mentally, that is – oh well, read some calming tales and generally, calm him down in every way. If he is calm, that is, does not show emotion in response to that phrase, but shows emotion in response to the statement: "The world is light", then the opposite actions need to be taken – tell him some stories mentally, vivid, unusual, so as to

15

achieve a certain level of mental excitement of the child. All this can be felt, that is, the child may show no external signs and the criterion of how he reacts will be your own opinion, including your mental opinion. That is, we are already talking about the telepathic level of communication. This way I have provided the telepathic level of communication, at which you can already say, concentrating on the first day of birth and on the entire stage of your work with the child, that the *Creator determined for him the task, and this task is creation and acquiring knowledge, and he must work on this task, helping himself in his development by active movements and already try to talk, mentally or by some other action, in the way he wants.* He must speak as logically as possible.

On the fifteenth day after birth, you need to show him the letter "A" mentally or in the form of a drawing, and say that; that is, in principle you can show him any letter, the first letter of an alphabet and say that *there is the letter, which has been created here in order to communicate. But he may communicate without letters.*

That means on the sixteenth day after birth it is necessary to tell him *about plants and animals, and that in the course of eternal life they will all have an infinite existence, such will be the conditions created on Earth in the world.*

On the seventeenth day after birth, it will be necessary to tell the child that *the world is set up in a very large space where it is located; the configuration of the world is infinite and the spaces are very large.*

On the eighteenth day after birth, it is necessary to mentally tell the child that *as the world is very large, in order to travel in it the concept of time is required, that so it goes with the world, when you move around it, it takes time.*

On the nineteenth day after birth, it is necessary to tell the child that *frequently his only task will be ensuring creative building, and therefore he should learn from the start which mechanisms of that process he should master already now, starting from this day.*

On the twentieth day after birth, you must concentrate on the first and second day after birth along this axis which I have drawn, and try to convey the sensations and memories which were there on the first and second day mentally to the child. Even if you do not remember – concentrate, that is, so to speak, if you cannot recall the details, concentrate on the numbers one and two along this axis and take them and transfer them over, mentally, to the twentieth day and mentally convey to the child. That is, this way the work is already in progress for transferring thoughts by means of the system.

On the twenty-first day after birth, you need to clarify that *every element is reflected in the world by some type of scheme.* That is, the ray of light may have a shadow, a number may have a reflection, that is, the reverse, mirror number, or a number may simply be written or glued together, and it will also produce a shadow, but it will also be a number at the same time. There is no need to simplify the task – you need to explain it precisely the way I say. That is, if make a glued structure of number twenty-one and stand it up and illumine it with a ray of light, it will also produce a shadow. That is, not only the ray of light has a shadow, but it can also come from a number, and the number is a symbol, for example, of twenty-one objects. This way try to explain it in great detail, you can allocate quite a lot of time to that, say, up to half an hour of continuous mental contact, in order to explain that all phenomena are related to each other both symbolically and directly without the symbolic level.

On the twenty-second day after birth, that is, it is necessary to say that there are *real connections behind the symbols, which frequently cannot be seen after the symbol has already been shown; they are not visible at once and the child must have an understanding of them. He must feel his well being, he must be able to cope with some feelings, with some possible deviations in his health – on his own. Because this is how he was created, originally. It is imperative that this be explained – that he has been so crea-ted, forever healthy, and therefore he already has a mechanism for coping.* That is, this is similar to a persuasive conversation that an adult has, that is, with someone whom he is nurturing. That is, here another action needs to be performed on the twenty-second day. Along a line drawn from number twenty return along the vector to the first day after birth and immediately from there return to number twenty. That is, perform mentally this discreet, that is, disjointed level of following the thought, that is, from the twentieth to the first, and from the first to the twentieth day.

After having done the work on the twenty-second day after birth, that is, it is followed by the twenty-third day after birth, that is, where you will tell to your child that *he must be capable of communicating with small child-ren like himself – mentally, while they are located in completely different areas of the planet, and may even be located in different points in time. This will not be a stopping point for him – he can still contact those same children who are also twenty-three days old, or when you were twenty-three days; and show him the specific practices.* Imagine when you were twenty-three days old and try to join with your child at the level of tele-pathy, that is, mentally imagine yourself as small and located as if next to him, listening to him there, holding him close, then you will feel how he is communicating with you, in what language and what symbols he uses and it will become clearer to you; the language in which you communicate may become very varied, and then you will be already in a position to convey very quickly all the creative knowledge which you have accumulated. That

18

is, it is such a powerful day with respect to transferring all the knowledge you have accumulated, – either instantaneously as one impulse, or in parts, with detailed batches.

On the twenty-fourth day after birth, you need to tell the child that *all numbers are united, and from numbers you can obtain again a simpler number.* So, for example, you could explain it that by adding two plus four and, turning it upside down, you will receive the number nine. That is, talk about that side of numbers.

On the twenty-fifth day after birth, you need to say that there, *turning everything the other way around and having thus obtained nine, that is turning upside down the two plus four, turning it around, we have nine, but as it turns out that two plus five is seven, but if we have on the left side two plus four upside down is nine, and two plus five is seven, that means we can obtain seven from nine, if we take that number two and subtract it.* That is, it is necessary to start performing mentally something like these types of calculations of that nature as I stated, but in such a way that he could add up numbers regardless of their locations. That is, not in the logical way, but the way I explain by rotating the symbols, or by the way of comparison; that if, for example, there is a number two next to a four, then in principle we will have two plus two which gives us four, but two through two – we receive a mirror reflection and can use that mirror reflection as subtraction; that is, the child must learn to subtract not what they teach them in those schools, but to subtract by combining the symbol with reality. That is, to work on the fabric of reality right away, and not on the symbolic basis, which is a reflection of reality. More precisely, if this were to be explained, then, as I explained two plus four, it should be six, through turning around, that is the physical turnaround that occurs, in physical reality, for example, if we cut out a figure six, we will have a nine;

two plus five is seven, and we will be able to obtain that seven if we take the two out of the nine, the two that was there in the number two plus four, for example. So, but in fact it should be two plus seven, so it goes that the four here played the role of the seven, had it not been turned around, but when we turned it upside down then it started to play the role of seven, that is, you need to say that the numbers may be added and transformed in this manner. And this way it is possible to develop any systems of one's own, detailing the world, showing that through connections it can be made most unusual, most colorful and at that stage this is a great pleasure. The same kind of work could be performed not necessarily with numbers, but with some objects. For example, there is an object nearby, there is a TV set and the baby's bed, even though they may be in different rooms. Tell him to move them mentally so as to place the TV set in front of himself and watch different programs. What he sees inside is a symbol, and what the TV set shows is reality. Mental transfer is also a symbol, but he, through a symbolic transfer, obtains reality. This is the training that needs to be performed with the child on day twenty-five.

On the twenty-sixth day after birth, you need to convey to the child that *he is already a grown adult person and must look at himself in the future, where he is a grown adult person.* When he looks, he must immediately arrange it so that all is well for him there, if he, well, thinks, that something needs to be improved there, in the future. For that you also should try to mentally look where your child looked or wants to look, and also try to improve the situation there, that he has in the future where he is a grown adult person.

On the twenty-seventh day after birth, you need to say that this is *again number nine, but this time it does not need to be turned upside down if they are combined, that is, if you add two plus seven. Or if you superimpose two and seven.* That is, explain in the way that you find more convenient.

On the twenty-eighth day after birth, tell the child *about your parents, that there are connections in existence that are biological and hereditary, that there are very many people, who are called relatives, acquaintances and friends,* that they will have to interact and this way you should try that the child make as many sounds as possible on that day, so that he would communicate mostly using words – that is, singing some songs, moving actively.

On the thirtieth day after birth, try to engage more in physically active movements, that is, explain that *he should walk; it is possible to work on that mentally, and mentally perform movements; it is necessary to provide more physical massage, for example, and try to say to him that he should help his parents, he should develop, he will have to do a lot of physical work for himself and therefore his task is physical development – as active as possible, but it must be – and that is the most important part in all this explanation – infinite. That is, he should develop based on infinite physical development.* The way I explained it, all these actions can be performed with any person, at any stage of his life. Simply it is necessary to mentally enter those days after his birth and do the same thing that one would do with an actual newborn; therefore, it is clear that this system makes it possible to restore the physical health of a person.

That is, on the thirty-first day after birth, you need to say that the *world is arranged both in a uniform and diverse way at the same time.* That is, for example, if you were to take a cube, or a ball, or a plant – they are in the form of separate elements, but within the plant there are leaves, within the cubes there are sides, and if the cubes were to be joined, there would be two cubes with sides touching; as a result, if they were to be glued, there would be a parallelepiped, and so it goes that a lot of phenomena may be created in the world, of which already by that time the child may be aware, as of very diverse phenomena.

Therefore, what was said with respect to each day for the newborn matters for one's own transfer of telepathic thoughts for each day and, correspondingly, development of one's own methods. Further on I will provide information for each month after birth starting from the day of birth, with respect to each month, starting from the second one, that is, – during the first month there were days from day one to day thirty-one. That is, it will be followed by the second month, the third month etc. up until the twelfth month, and then it will be after the configuration by months and days for the duration of one year, there will be the second year, the third year, etc. up to seven years inclusive. After that it will be broken down by periods.

This way during the second month, that is, after birth, you need to mentally convey to the child that *light consists of different hues of light. That if more light is combined, it may not necessarily become brighter from that, but it may simply have different colors.* This way you need to convey during the second month already information about colors, and that having data on colors it is possible to give a specific color to every event; then, based on the concentration of colors and how they are mixed, a newborn baby could already orient himself in that information and control it.

During the third month, that is, it is necessary to convey to the child mentally that *he has arms, legs, a body, and they are connected in this way, and that he has a head, so, in general, all the body parts; that if one, that is, develops them constantly, then they will become indestructible, and this is the way it is necessary to convey these thoughts, so that he would understand how necessary it is to do that.* That is, it needs to be regarded from his point of view. The main thing here is that to look, mentally that is, at his palms, so, look at the palms, for example, of the child to men-

22

tally convey, that is, that at that moment this palm, that is, in the form of your thought – it transitions into his thinking, that is, he is supposed to see himself as if through your thought. Then he will already begin to develop the body in infinity.

During the fourth month, that is, it is necessary to convey mentally to the child that *he must be able to read, write and walk. But he should be able to do all that on his own originally.* That is, you should try to explain to him specifically that he should do it himself, and later, when others teach him, he should only compare it to what they are teaching him and try, that is, what he is being taught and try to correct what he has learnt.

During the fifth month, the child needs to learn about the *concept of infinite and finite. Infinity...*

During the fifth month, it is necessary to give the child knowledge about what infinite and finite are. Infinity – you will need to explain mentally, encompassing the infinite world, or by spreading your arms and showing, that there is where infinity is, it is big, while the concept of finite – there you bring your hands together to one point and say to the child, that *he must think in the same way mentally, that every object consists of an infinite and a finite part; for the explanation of those two parts show the specific outline of an object and even try to find, for example, in each object some infinite outline and a finite one and this way you transition to writing, where you explain each letter, each word, each element, which you want to explain using that same position.*

During the sixth month, it is necessary to provide knowledge on what is *development and movement; that life is an infinite value, and in the finite form it is manifested in the form of a body.* That is, the body is not the end, that is, but the beginning of an infinite life, and during that try to orient the child so that his education would go through continuous contact with you.

You must at all times feel the spiritual world of the child, strive to ensure that the spiritual picture of the world that he has is harmonious with the entire environment.

During the seventh month, the child must understand *that all things are connected, that when he eats he receives energy, food, and that is why he can walk; when he thinks he can receive the same thing or he can produce food.* That is, he must be sensitized to the fact, that receiving food is a process connected with his spirit. That this is provided by God and at the same time this is spirit and this is provided by parents. He must see all those connections and have his own attitude to everything. Attitude of harmony, attitude of control, relations of these connections, when all these phenomena bring him a good feeling, feeling of harmony.

During the eighth month, it is necessary to explain to the child that *when events occur in the world, these events are always relevant to him. That it is necessary to regard the events that happen in such a way as to harmonize them, so that the events are positive for everybody; that is, try to demonstrate that everything that happens outside of him is still always connected to him.* This can be explained telepathically or using examples.

During the ninth month, it is necessary to explain *the origin of letters from sounds.* That is, to describe it so – that each letter may signify a sound, and each and every symbol may signify some information; that is you have to try to make sure that the child, that is, would understand where the information is presented in symbolic form and what is the essence, meaning of information: it may be symbolic or it may be true, but through the symbolic system it is possible to control the meaning; for example, write letters – there will be a word, etc.

During the tenth month, it is necessary to try to show the child *through telepathy or on the physical level that when he is looking far ahead using physical vision, then he can, using more long-distance vision than the physical one, see the same thing, but from the other side.* That is, in practice, you will mentally visualize it for him, that he is looking somewhere along a straight line, and you look as if facing him, mentally, showing that over there, that is, one can see. This is already the development of clairvoyance.

During the eleventh month, you should show the *system of forecasting,* that is, the system of controlling projection, when what he sees moving from afar, towards him or away from him – these are controllable forecast values. That is, he must understand that everything that he is regarding in the world and everything that he can see ahead and everything which he is preparing: to eat in the morning, for example, or watching a movie or studying letters – all this is controllable and he can learn in advance how to do it better. Attune him in this way for every day, so that he would look at each following day, the future time, and would try to be most useful for all and for himself in the direction, also, of saving of the world, that is, would try to organize his actions, mental and physical.

During the twelfth month, it is necessary to show the child that *when we touch finite objects at the physical level it is possible to obtain an infinite point.* For example, if you take a cube, touch a surface with one point of it and say: where the corner of the cube is touching the side of another cube, there is a very small point there – so small that it can be infinitely small; that is, demonstrate that finite objects create infinity.

And then, that is, there will already be next year and further on the methodology is broken down by year. That is, now the things which were said day by day during the first month, and then using methods designated for each month, that is – after that, within this system, they will be arranged by years.

That is, during the second year, it is necessary to show the child that

25

the *world is infinite in the same way as the possibility of vision, that is, transition to thinking.* That is, when the child is looking at the clouds – that is, at the air, at the horizon – it is possible to use vision, but it can be transferred to thinking, that is, thinking can become infinite as well. And since he can also see things that don't end, the finite outlines contain infinite spaces. And also it is necessary to explain to him that, that is, further on there is the infinity of his name, infinity of his thought, infinity of his connections, infinity of his friendship and love; and it needs to be shown, that all these concepts are related to the real infinity of the world. That is, education must be organic – not a formal explanation of infinity by itself, but the connection: that the infinity of the world brings about infinity of love. The infinity of the world with all stars and galaxies creates an infinity of relations, say, kindness to parents, kindness towards the world, towards constructive creation, that is, there is creation in the world, and also show that the child even needs to understand that on the basis of the physical vision. That is, for example, for a comparison of the way it happens, say: if one looks at the distance, the road ends there, one horizon there meets the other, for example, the horizon coming from the sea from the infinite plane; and finiteness brings about infinity at the point when they converge for physical vision; in the same way thoughts can provide infinity at the point where they are finite.

During the third year, it is necessary to educate the child with respect to those who are around him. He must know how to correct those around him, he must be able to stabilize the attitude of others who are close around him, and be able to spread this attitude onto everyone around. That is, for this you need to explain that each person is engaged in some relationships, that is, each event happens in accordance with certain laws; and the child's task is to sit there and control all those events in such a way that it would be good for everybody. For control you have to show him the following practice: to demonstrate that if you place your hand on a table or on a chair, for example – on a smooth surface – and spread the fingers, then there is a certain distance between the fingers. So, that distance represents all events, and the fingers are all the people whom he knows, sees and remembers; and it is possible to increase the number by several times, that is, one can imagine a lot of fingers; and so his task is to ensure that the distance – between the fingers, that is, – be good and proper so that the fingers are comfortable, so that all the people may be good, all people be arranged for goodness and kindness and develop creatively. In this manner he will just simply move his fingers about and exert control. Then, you need to say that it can be done mentally, it is not necessary to move the fingers even, it is possible to transmit at the mental level without showing it at the physical one.

During the fourth year, that is, it is necessary to show the child that *there is feedback for every phenomenon.* That is, for example, if he threw a stone into the water, and if it was a flat stone which would touch the water in several places and create waves, then the waves would touch as well and one wave would overlap with another, and if this stone were to skip over the surface of the water several times, the interaction of those waves may be at one point from the same stone touching the water at different times. And so it goes, that those who are under the water – fishes – could see it as well; and the waves touching each other, that is, there is feedback for every phenomenon, because the fishes, once they saw the stone and the waves, would swim away from the stone, for example, and during that time feedback would be expressed so that when the waves touched the fishes would see that as well, but this was at the same time as there were no fishes near that stone. That is, use this example to explain that there is a consequence for every event, and teach him control through consequences, that is, when some sign of an event is available to him, the child must understand that through this sign he can trace it to the cause: who had thrown the stone and in what way. This is called development of forecasting ability through clairvoyance, and in the future it will result in healing skills; that is, finding those connections enables one to find the cause and eliminate the disease. Also, already at that age it is possible to tell him that he can regenerate himself and others, and develop this ability in other people as well. There is a mandatory element: he must mentally transfer this knowledge to others.

During the fifth year, that is, it is necessary to explain to the child that the way world works is when everyone wishes for the development of the world, then the world will necessarily develop in this way, the good and positive way, and that he must also want that development – the positive creative development of the world. That is, he must want it this way, so that his action and wishes would encompass that. He must think in this way, so that the world would develop in the positive creative direction; and so it is necessary to work on these thinking methods, that is, demonstrate how one must think; for example, that look at oneself, that is, in this way since the whole world may be touching points, then just by moving or being in a good attitude of spirit it is possible to control this world moving it in the positive direction.

That is, during the sixth year of life, it is necessary to give the child knowledge regarding when he is going somewhere – when *he goes to some meeting, when he is being met there or not being met, when he does something, all this occurs in relation to the world that has already been created or being created, in connection with the Creator.* And when these meetings happen, he must see, where there are manifestations of the Crea-tor, where there are manifestations of the global picture of the world, where the fundamental, that is, the principal level of the world brings about adult life, that is, where the transition from action and from understanding of the world, that is, to the specific practice takes place in the form of information, that is, he must understand the fundamental meaning of the world which follows these specific actions. Explain it the way I said it using the level of examples of meetings, events, etc.

At the seventh year of life, the child must very clearly, in deterministic form convey how the event is set up from the standpoint of the fundamental level of the world. The fundamental level of the world you can explain on your own, take it from my lectures, or demonstrate using the very simplest examples. When a tree grows, it grows because there was, that is, the nutritive environment. And the nutritive environment is predicated by what is there in the earth. So, the earth is created, that is, by the Creator, as well as everything around is created by the Creator, and he must understand how the Creator created all this. Then he will have a system. In order for him to have a system he must understand the connections – that everything that was created by the Creator, that is, could be created as well, and then it will be correct. When he understands that, he will develop in school in terms of learning to read and developing any skills, in harmony with the creative idea which the Creator, that is, set forth in the form of the creation of the world.

This way I have completed here, in this lecture, the first period of development of the child: up to seven years of age. Now there is the second period of development of a person, which is from age eight till fourteen.

That is, when he is eight, that is, you need to convey *knowledge in the form of presenting literature at the telepathic level, etc.,* that is, to the person regarding the fact that the world is discrete, that is, each part of the world may be independent, and that it is possible to find connections between the elements of the world and obtain completely new solutions, that is, this is the principle of searching for new solutions. Generally speaking, in this development it is always possible to go back and in hindsight telepathically explain to any child or explain it all to a child, located at any distance that anything can be done mentally, that anything can be done physically in parallel.

That is, during the ninth year it is necessary to give the child *the mechanism for specific practices, specific tasks, when he would be able to tie all the phenomena of reality in the form of control;* that is, he must receive a very clear controlling structure, he must understand that the world is controllable, he must use that and have a very clear, harmonious so to speak, smooth methodology. He must feel that this is the same as modeling clay, which you can shape in different ways and obtain different outlines; this should be based on the impressions and this should be the action in reality. To achieve that it is necessary to practice more with some accepted physical realities, with some fundamental practices and attempt to show that from the standpoint of the fundamental reflection of the world, one can do everything using one's consciousness and it is not necessary to do it physically.

During the tenth year, that is, within the tenth year of life the child must *understand the essence of combining the elements which are part of living nature with the elements, that is, which are different by nature; and in this case the essence stems from the common goal of both types of elements.* You would say that a tree is growing so as to provide oxygen to people; say that the soil is there so that people would walk on it. That is, as it would seem a living tree generates oxygen and the soil also exists for the purpose of generating life. That is, it needs to be shown that in principle everything is moving in the direction of life; prove this by illustrating with specific

30

practical examples from the practical experience of the child.

During the eleventh year of life, it is necessary to explain to the child that when *he develops creatively and progressively, he is building for himself a firm systematic future, and this is accounted for by the fact that such development is always associated with accumulating knowledge;* show on specific examples that he is studying some science, some subject – he is capable of working telepathically, he can exert control, and creative activity brings about new horizons for creation. That is, only creation is the principle of universal development, including development of the child himself. He should not destroy anything.

At twelve years of age, it is necessary to show the child that *he is, in fact, already an adult person,* it is just that before, that is, he was looking at everything from the standpoint of development, which already brings him to the adult state, and his preceding development was in no way different from the development which will occur in the adult state. That is, what is called adult at the age of twelve needs to be accumulated and concentrated as a combined point, where there is no disconnect between the preceding age and subsequent age. That is, at twelve the child must become aware that he is the same as, let's put it that way, all other creative elements of reality and that he has an infinite future, that he is light and happy, that everything will always be good for him. And for that it is necessary to, let's put it that way, congratulate him more, provide more presents, and try to make the image of the world consist exclusively of light.

At thirteen, the child must understand absolutely clearly that *by using intellectual concentration, by using the fact that he can properly concentrate, behave correctly at the level of thought – he can rule the world, rule reality,* and for this, that is, he must understand that this is precisely the age, when, that is, those actions would be quite acceptable; that is, that is,

31

those actions would be feasible, those actions would be necessary for him. And he must very clearly react to the fact that thought changes reality. He must, that is, make sure of that in a certain way and attempt to behave in such a way that his thoughts are very specific and he already needs to treat thoughts as a control mechanism.

At fourteen years of age, that is, so it goes, that the child who is growing up, that is, I am going to call him now an adult person; so, at fourteen it is necessary to convey to the person information, that the *world can be changed according to his thinking.* So the way he thinks is the way the Creator helps his development, that is, he must feel an organic connection with the Creator. He must feel him clearly and strive so that his actions on a spiritual basis are in line with information that the Creator, that is, desires from that person.

This way the second period comprises years eight, nine, ten, eleven, twelve, thirteen, and fourteen.

Now for the third period. It is characterized by the fact that it is going to be used in the infinite future, cycles but by adding the subsequent coefficient, literally, by number. That is, for example, if we are talking about starting from twenty-two, then, it will be the same information, that is, as for fifteen years of age, but by concentrating on number four, etc.

That is, for the age of fifteen, it is important that the person *perceive reality as very specific control and completely methodological, with some specific methods and generalized consequences.* That is, he must see that the specific has a generalized nature, that from the general it is possible to arrive at the specific; he must understand that out of any small sign it is possible to see a major consequence or a major past. At fifteen he must control the future in such a way as to make the future be arranged and disposed, that is, towards him.

At sixteen, the child must, or rather at sixteen the person must understand the truth that life is a principle; that is, at в sixteen the child must become aware and know that *the principle of life is the mental understanding of the time-space from the standpoint of data, which he had at twelve, ten, or even earlier, as early as three years of age.* That is, he must look at time and space as at a structure with which he is already familiar and to which he can relate. This relation should not change. He must just feel the growth of his body, growth of his mind and this sensation, this feeling should serve as a platform for having infinite development. At sixteen he must fully see the infinity of his development.

At seventeen, the person must *approach the essence of God as an implementation of the idea of a person within eternal life.* He must understand that his life and development are this sequence of events which are determined by God; that he in conjunction with these events is a god-creative personality and is striving towards the Creator in his actions, and that his actions must be thought through, that his actions of the deification of life, of striving towards eternal life must be technology-based and he must understand that, and then the application methodologies which he will be using for control will be quite specific and will be based on the specific practice that the child has, that is, which the young man has, the adult has – that is, it is necessary to use all the practice in order to bring about the event – all the practice available.

At eighteen, that is, the person must understand that when an event occurs, then he is fully responsible for that event, that is, if he believes that he is responsible for this event. That is, here strengthening of his personal opinion must take place, but on the general scale of things he must understand that he is in any case connected with the event at the level of general connections, and here it is necessary to develop the moral criterion, when he reacts to this event from the standpoint of general connections, that he is a participant, working on the principle of self-governance and on the basis that this touches him personally in a deep way. That is, as for the depth of the soul, depth of the spirit – it is necessary to understand it on the basis of the specific events and control them based on the moral control principles, which in terms of political levels have the same levels of creation as life in society does, in human society or any other.

At the age of nineteen, the person should clearly, that is, *imagine, or even clearly know all future events at the level of their connections, at the level of their outcomes and, depending on the purpose, shape the ideology of behavior.* That is, he must, as it happens, do everything, taking into account a completely clear beacon and a very precise level of knowledge, which is sometimes latent and intuitive, and sometimes it is absolutely clear that a person possesses it.

At the age of twenty, the person must strive to become aware of reality in this way – that reality can always be controlled. That is, no matter what events might have occurred, reality can always be transformed in the way the person wants. Therefore he may be calm and certain; he must carry forth light, he must bring forth intelligence, he must bring forth good, and when he stands on that, he will always be ahead, he will always be winning, he will always be successful and will always be a beacon for all those who follow the same line, that is, of mutual movement forward and upward, which is to lead to universal well-being; and he must understand this, that he is coming to the situation when a lot of information having to do with the development of people depends on his actions.

At twenty-one, a person must know that *all the future must, that is, be implemented within the timeline which he set earlier.* Infinite future has infinite deadlines, therefore he must strive to accomplish that technologically. That is, this is the year when actions begin. The person must know that the year when he begins to act is the year which brings him to infinity; even though this is true with respect to each preceding year, but this year moves him along the path of infinity significantly faster. This way it is possible to increase the rate of speed of adapting the spirit to infinite development, that is, by concentrating on how that is achieved at twenty-one.

That is, the following periods are practically the same as the third period, that is, the one from fifteen till twenty-one, and the only thing is that it is necessary to concentrate in each period respectively on the number of the period itself. For example, how about the forth period? This is the one from the age of twenty-two and so it goes till the age of twenty-nine. That is, if we want to talk about development, for example, at the age of twenty-two years, then it is necessary to concentrate on number four and develop the same things as is suggested for development at the age of fifteen. That is, in fact, twenty-two, twenty-three, twenty-four, twenty-five, twenty-six, twenty-seven, and twenty-eight – it is up to twenty-eight years, inclusive. So it goes that the third period, the fourth period – the fourth period covers the age of up to and including twenty-eight. Which includes twenty-two, twenty-three, twenty-four, twenty-five, twenty-six, twenty-seven, twenty-eight, and so, as I already explained, in order, that is, to concentrate on twenty, in order to develop at twenty-two years of age it is necessary to concentrate on the same things, that you, that is, were developing at the age of fifteen, but concentrating on the number of the period while doing that. Accordingly, for twenty-eight it covers the things that need to be developed at twenty-one, but while doing so it is imperative to concentrate on number four, when you think about it and develop in this direction. Accordingly, if we, that is, – and I will just use it for the sake of example – if we were to use the fifth period, which would already be twenty-nine, thirty, thirty-

35

one, thirty-two, thirty-three, thirty-four, thirty-five; that is, up to thirty-five years inclusive. That is, you need to simply concentrate on number five. That is, for the age of twenty-nine you concentrate on number five, and act in the same way as you are studying the same things that you did at fifteen in accordance with the same principles; but for thirty-five you concentrate on number five, – these are the same principles that were used for the age of twenty-one. So this is a kind of infinite system; that is, accordingly, if we are talking about the next period which is thirty-six, thirty-seven, thirty-eight, thirty-nine, forty, forty-one, forty-two; then it will be the same as, that is, at the age of thirty-six – at thirty-six one needs, that is, further on at thirty-six it means it is necessary at thirty-six to concentrate on the same thing, which means, that is, to develop the same aspects as for the age of fifteen in the first place, let's put it this way, and then concentrate on the level, the number of the period. And therefore so it goes that this way it is possible to develop infinitively with this system of number-based concentration. But this system, number-based concentration, it has another special aspect, in that when you concentrate on the same number it is still possible to make the numbers more varied. That is, numbers may be added up – four can be converted into two plus two, five can be converted into two plus three and then perform concentration through these numbers. Then other fine tints of numbers. How do you receive the guiding shades of meaning through number? The thing is that the principle here is simple, for example, concentrating on methodology, which is presented here for up to the age of fifteen, that is, you can accordingly, that is, develop completely new methodologies by breaking up the number there: for example, number is the period, it is number four, but the resulting idea during the concentration on number four has a fourfold increase, for example, a fourfold amplification, etc.. That is, each number may be used either as amplification, or as broadening, or as detailing by four times, that is, it is possible to do the same thing, say, through assigning to the number some forms of meaning.

That is, education at this level, for this cycle of education can be performed for any person, at any age, mentally transferring this education either onto oneself, or any other person. This way it is possible to develop the structure for practically any person and by doing so restore them spiritually, develop them spiritually and even cure of illnesses, etc. That is, this is practically education which is at the same time a universal control system, which can be, that is, either used directly, that is, in fact, you must regard the connections in such a way that these connections would lead to specific results in the real world. Here is a person, for example, and his situation is such that he must or wants to study in accordance with my system of educationя; then he would have to do it either in real time, or it is possible to do it from any time point, and even for an age higher than his own. That is, in fact it is possible to optimize the future this way. That is, using a specific example – if one were to take a specific example it would mean the following. For example, there is a person of a certain age. Let's say that he is, for example, eighteen; then he can, first of all, – if he had never previously encountered this system of education of mine, – do it all for himself, practically, to transmit to himself all these thoughts, which are set forth here, that is, starting from the state preceding birth. That is, secondly, he can do that with respect to any persony from negative infinity to positive infinity. That is, he can do it for a grandfather, for younger relatives, for friends of the older and younger ages, etc. That is, it is also certainly possible to work in real time. For each level, – that is for each year, for each principle he can develop the methodology on his own from the standpoint of those methods which I offer and principles which he obtains independently. That is, the development of a methodological basis can take any form; the most important thing is to adhere to the main direction of the methodology in those cases. If, for example, it is necessary to quickly learn a foreign language, if it is necessary to receive education in accordance with the harmonies of the world, in accordance with the creative building of the world, to rethink and review one's past education in accordance with the fundamental laws of the world, it is possible to use this system, adapting it for the knowledge you already have, or using the knowledge together, or selecting something, or just using this system of education as a single system, etc. That is, having a well-developed spirit, having the capacity to receive information, it is not necessary to use books in order to learn to exert control – it is possible to study independently and have all the answers, all the symbols, that is possible to know in advance, and the capacity for materialization enables one to obtain everything, up to the tests already written. That is, therefore what is implied by education here is the kind of education when the soul can build around it the necessary sequence of events, and those events are associated with numbers, that is, they are oriented towards the state of the soul itself. In practice, this system of education can be used to treat diseases. For example, if while learning to understand some system harmonious connections were not taken into account, that is, the fundamental nature of organization of knowledge or actions, then as part of overcoming some information in education cells may be changed, that is, there may be some diseases, and through clarification, telepathic transmissions to oneself or someone else it is possible to recover from illnesses. That is, if we are talking about events – it is possible to improve the event through harmonization of one's understanding, one's viewpoints with respect to the world, to one's development. That is, one's own development in this case will serve as the criterion of control, and the normalization of one's own development provides proper control

38

even in case you later do not perform specific technological actions to obtain a specific result. For example, if you need to pass a test, perform some action, receive some good event; so then you can affect the event itself, that is, by obtaining it, or simply bring to the harmonious norm, that is, in harmony with the surrounding world through education according to the system which I have now shown you, that you are your own information, that is, – then your event will in any case be positive for you. That is, according to this formation of events, including the restoration of one's own health and the health of others – is the correct orientation in the world of information, the correct understanding of the laws of the world, the correct understanding of the laws of the universe. And this education provides the capacity to have such understanding, it provides a capacity for original knowledge as to why the world is organized in this way, why things happen this way in the world, why events are connected to each other in this way and not some other way, and makes it possible to find new connections, develop one's own methodologies and systems of redemption and move along the infinite way of infinite life in the physical world, that is, and in the spiritual world and in the moral world as well. During this special moral laws of education may arise; education is the impetus which provides eternal stability. Correct education means stability forever; it is the idea of God. Because the Creator – God – he created the world, so that through understanding and knowledge of this world people would develop with respect to his idea of eternity; that is, education is in practice what you receive and see in front of yourself. Because when you do something and perform it – this is at the same time your education. Therefore, if you regard education as formation of the event from the standpoint of the fundamental level of the world you will then always have an instrument of control, and your education will be systemic and will not contain unexpected components that are unneeded, or some actions that are not needed for you. Therefore, when I speak about education, I mean that this education must, that is, having created a systematic level of favorable development, a systematic level of optimizing development, when you are in harmony with a continuously developing world, understand its connections and attempt to concurrently also develop the world in the direction of universal happiness, creative development, and then you arrive at the action already in the future as a known value. This is the method of how knowledge of the future is generated – the knowledge of the future which enables us, first of all, to be prepared for some events, and second, to control those events. In fact education is forming true information about the future, which will enable you to have the status which you have selected due to your original nature and essence and education from the standpoint of knowledge of fundamental connections, and ensures that true individuality which was inherently granted to you by the Creator. Education is your individuality. You receive what the Creator provided in the form of thought, in the form of information, in the form of development. When you see how he provided that, in accordance with which laws education has been built into your perception, when it forms in this context in connection with that, you obtain a complete personality, that true personality for which you are always striving in accordance with the design of God. The individual who receives a proper education, harmonious education, education with a knowledge of the fundamental laws of the world – that individual will already be developing in accordance with the laws bestowed upon it by the Creator. That is, it will be true development of personality and, having reviewed the process of the formation of everything in the world in terms of spiritual and physical from the standpoint of the objectives of the Creator, you obtain true development of information, you receive true knowledge of deep subjects in the world, deep reasons in the world, not only from the standpoint of some sciences, not only from the standpoint of some relative elements, but from the standpoint of maximum, the only one truth for you, from the standpoint of your whole personality which is following the design of the Creator into eternal existence, eternal life, towards immortality, when immortality is a reflection of the idea of the Creator, reflection of true knowledge of the Creator. In this way you, receiving a true and proper education, based on a fundamental level of knowledge of the world, which means also control over this world at the level of organization of the world of information, that is, and control of any part of the world, you receive, that is, the level which, in accordance with the initial idea, is that of the free and independent personality that was given to you by the Creator.

Grigori Grabovoi

Educational System of Grigori Grabovoi

For further information on the contents of this book contact:

SVET centre, Hamburg, Germany,

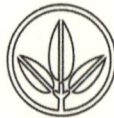

www.svet-centre.eu

Jeletzky publishing, Hamburg 2011

NOTES